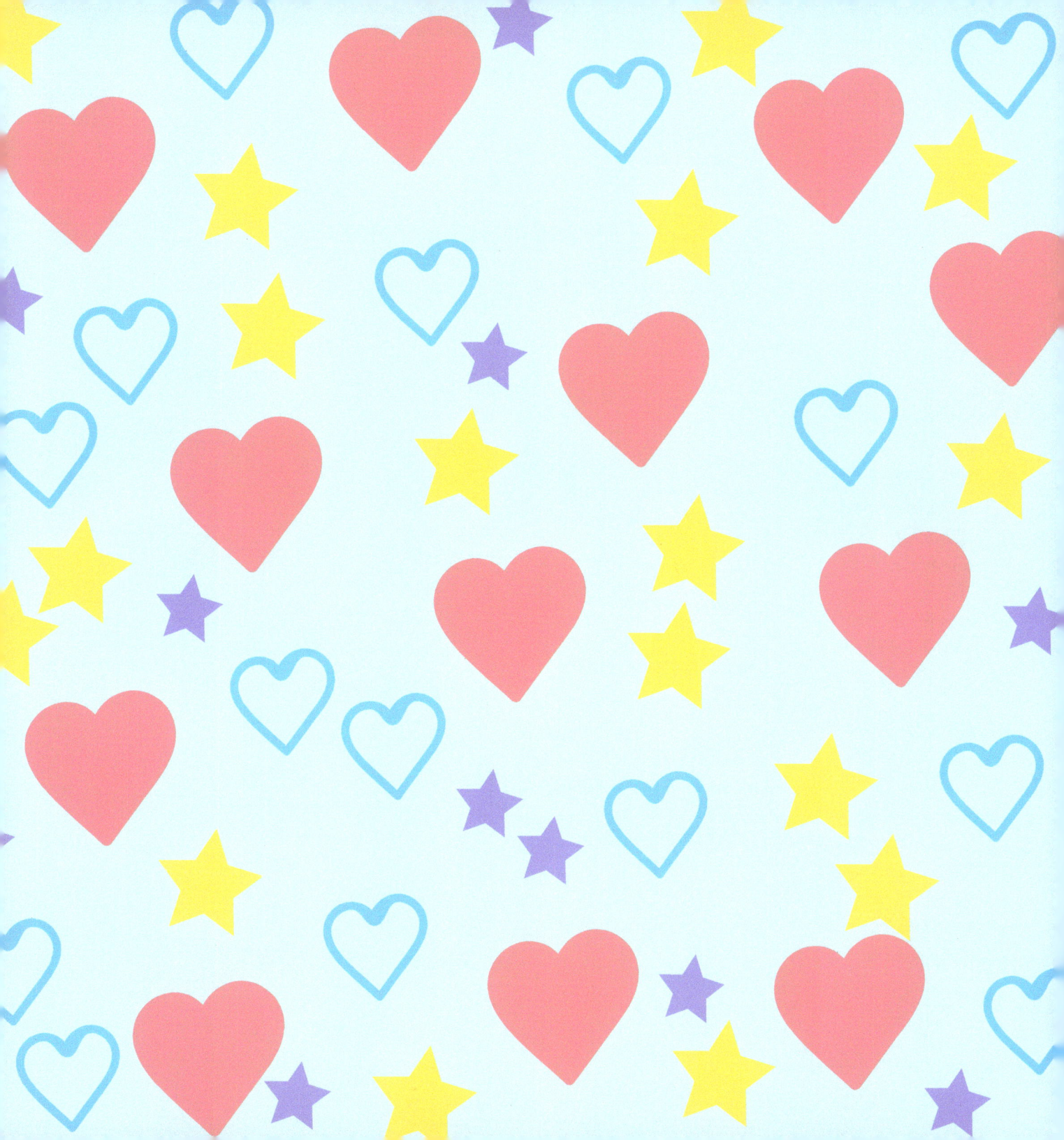

To all the Medical Mamas out there.

You are not alone. I see you x

Medical Mama

Written and Illustrated
by Lisa McArthur-Collins

First Printing 2024

Published by Little Wings Publishing
www.littlewingspublishing.com

ISBN 978-1-7635634-3-8 Paperback Version
ISBN 978-1-7635634-4-5 Hardcover Version

Medical Mama

by Lisa McArthur-Collins

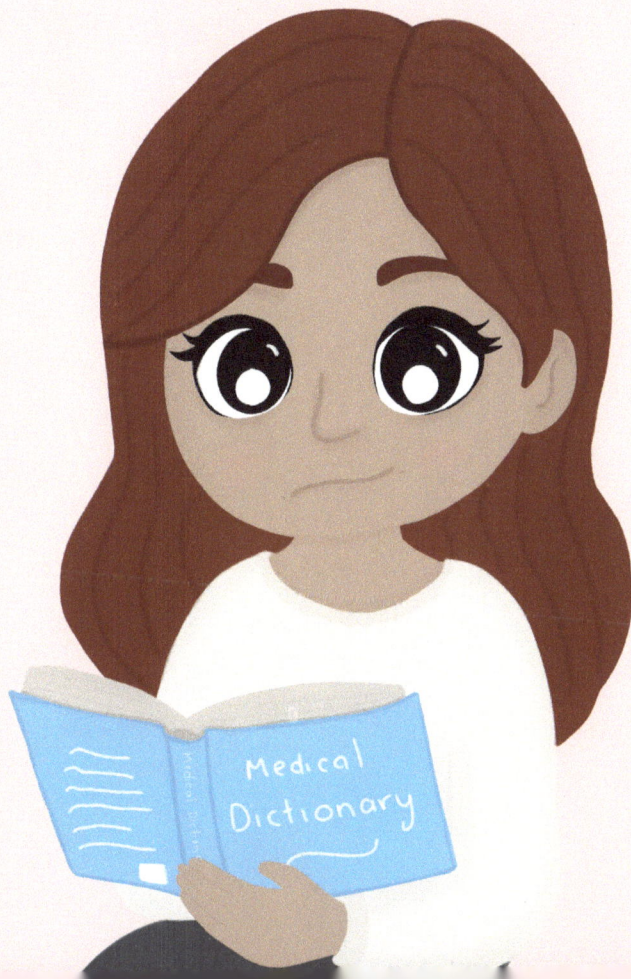

I see you,

Medical Mama.

I know it's hard.

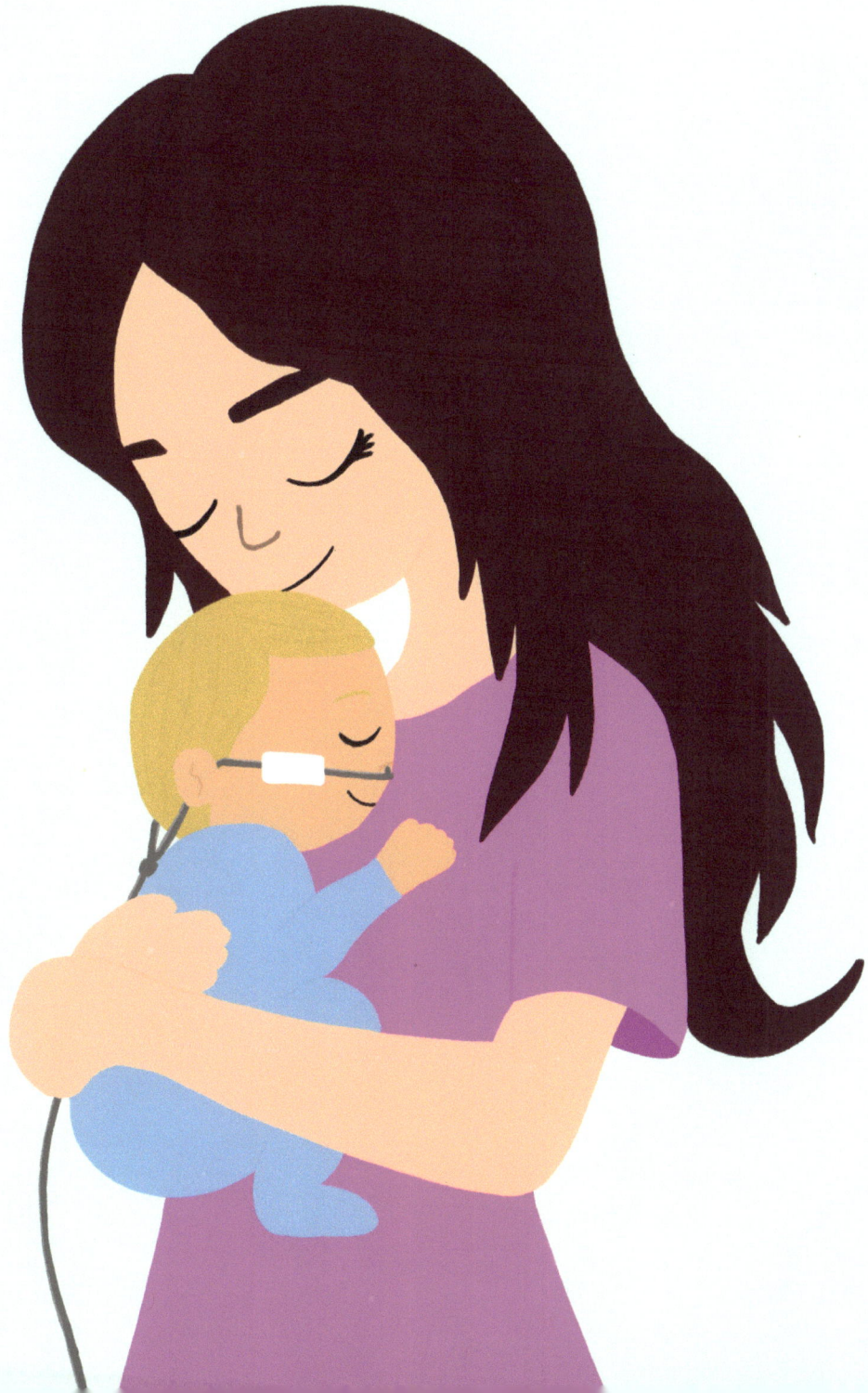

How you fight for
your little one,

Medical Mama,

doesn't go unnoticed.

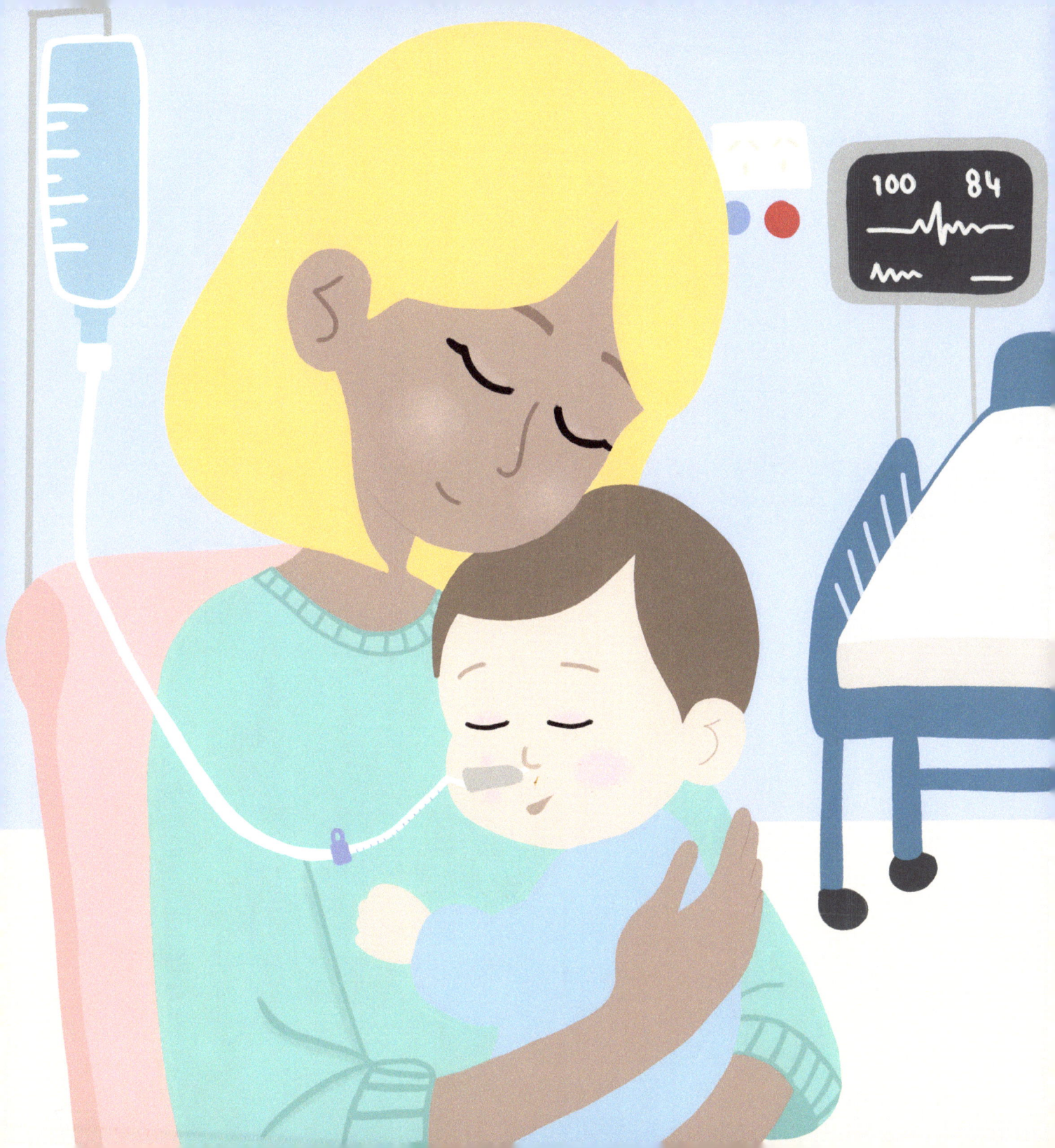

You wish your weeks were full of coffee dates and playground hangs.

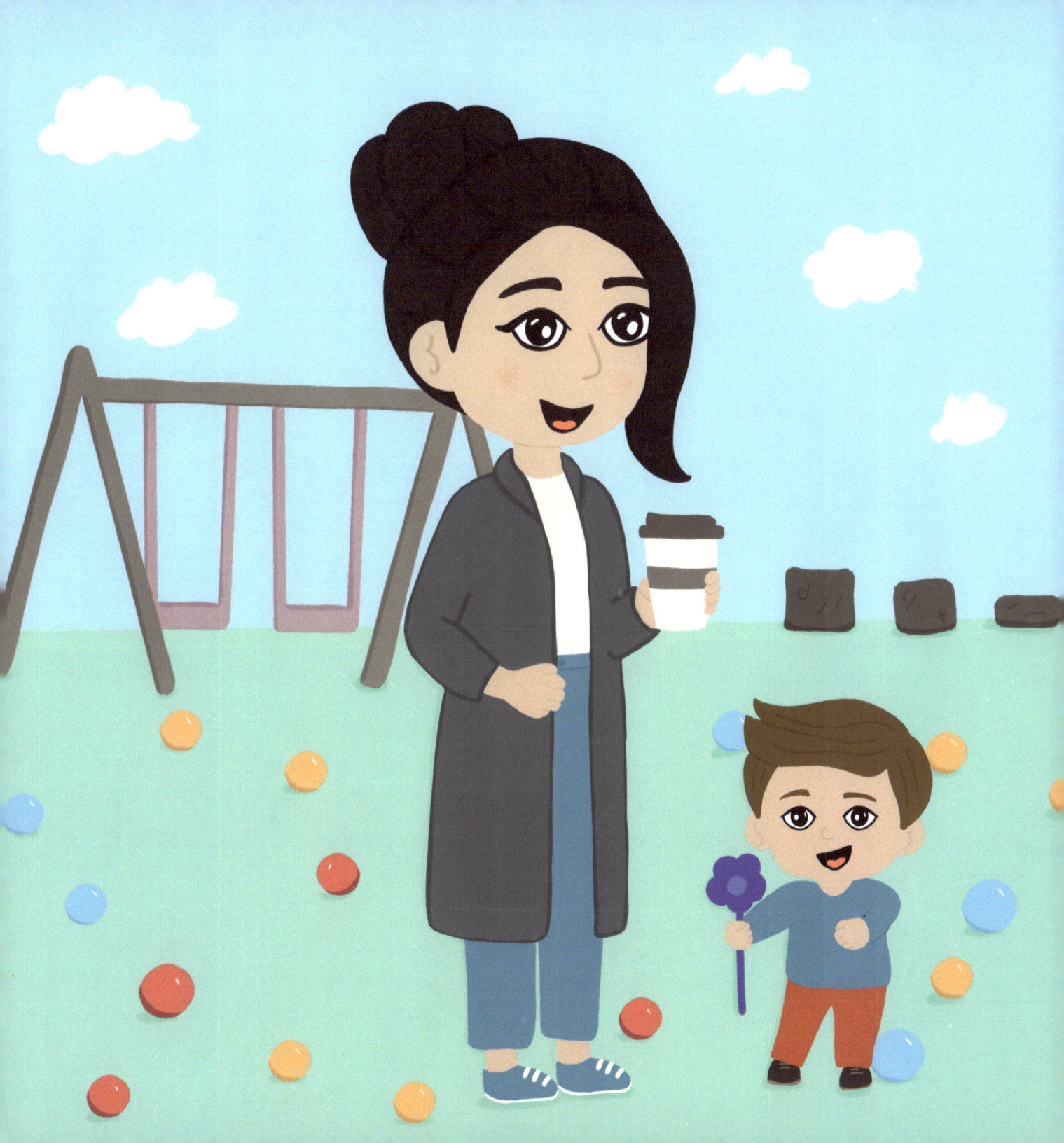

But instead, they're full of appointments and therapy sessions.

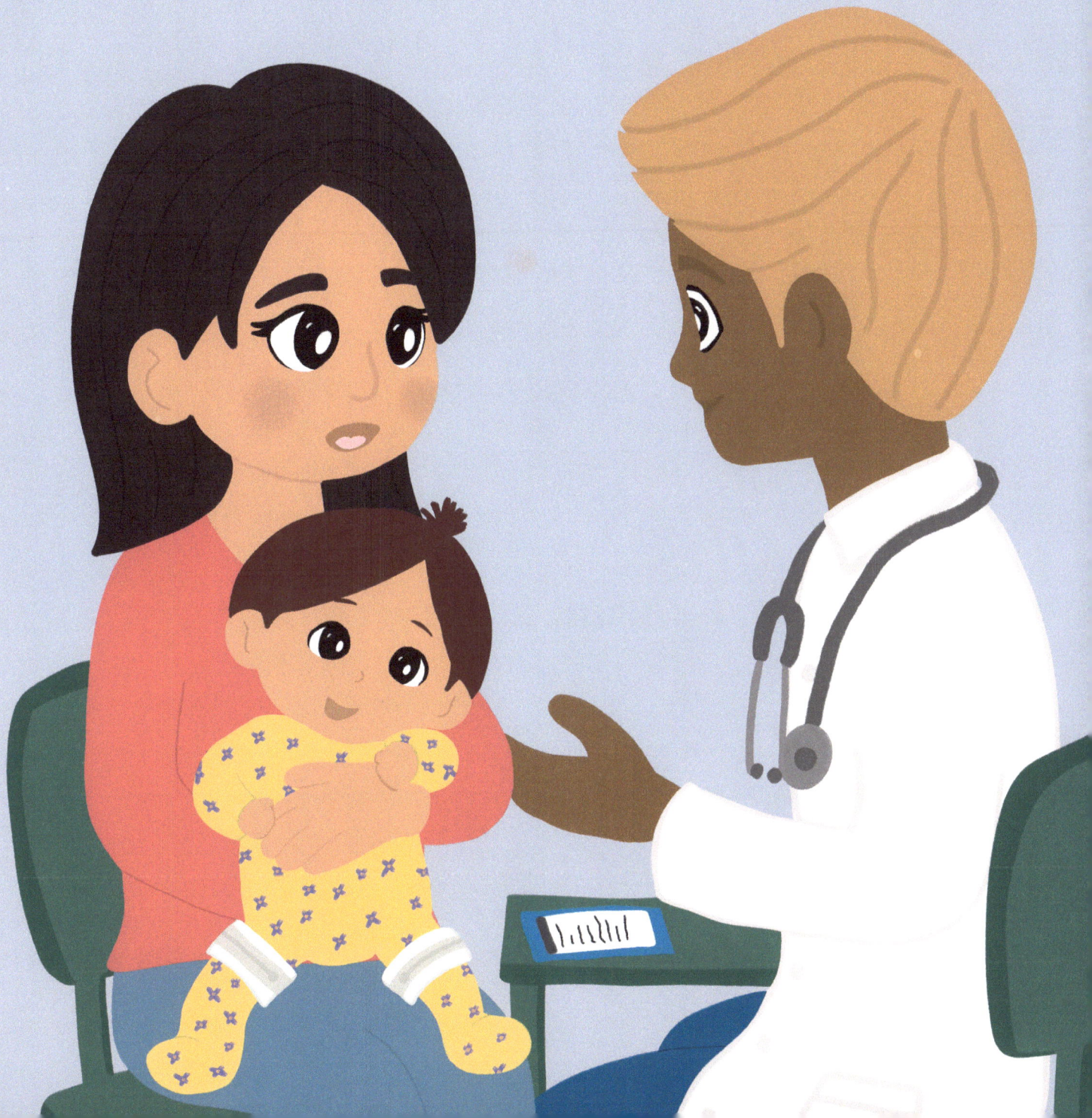

You frequent the cafe at the hospital more than any other.

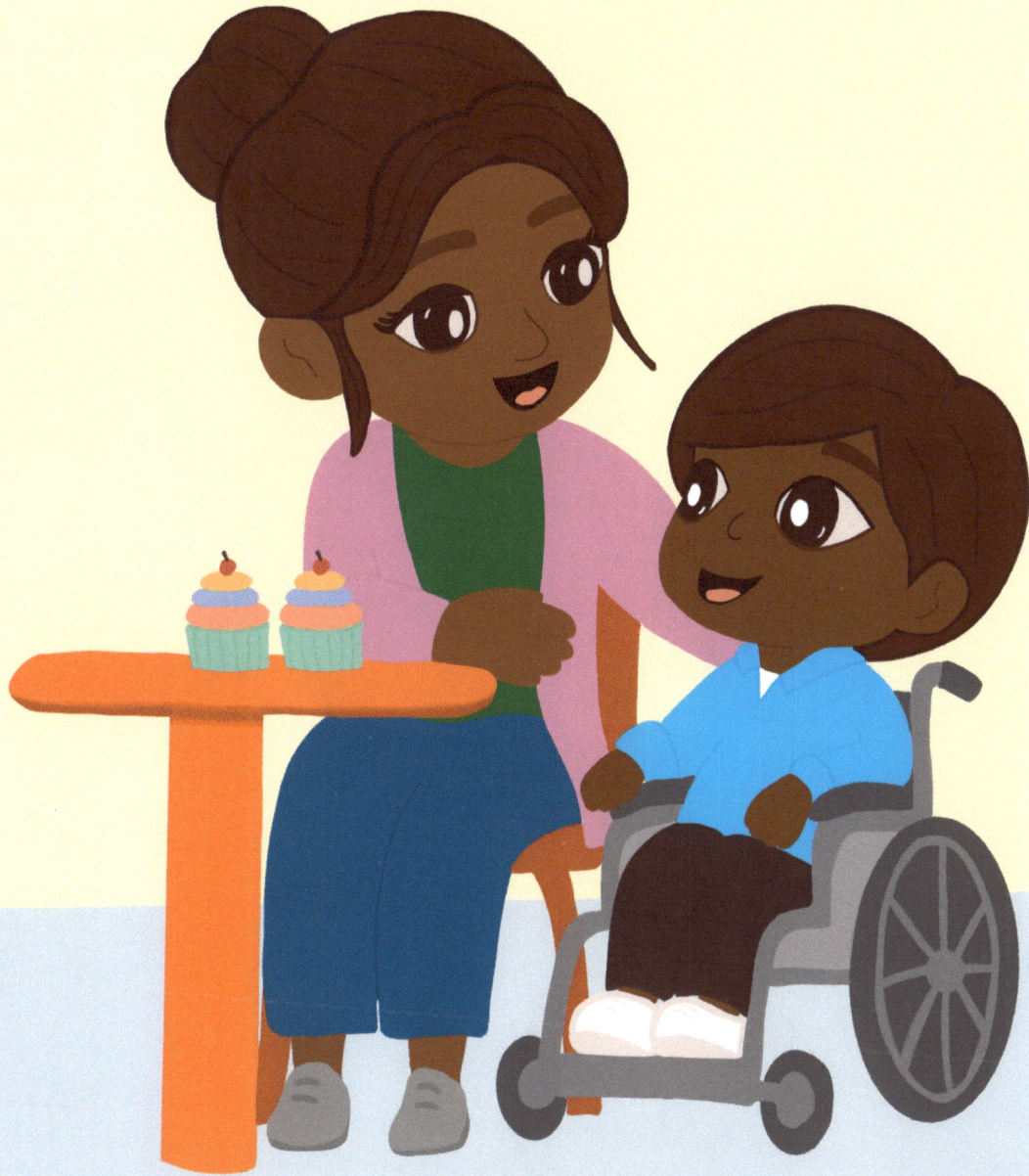

The list of medical terms you've learnt is forever growing.

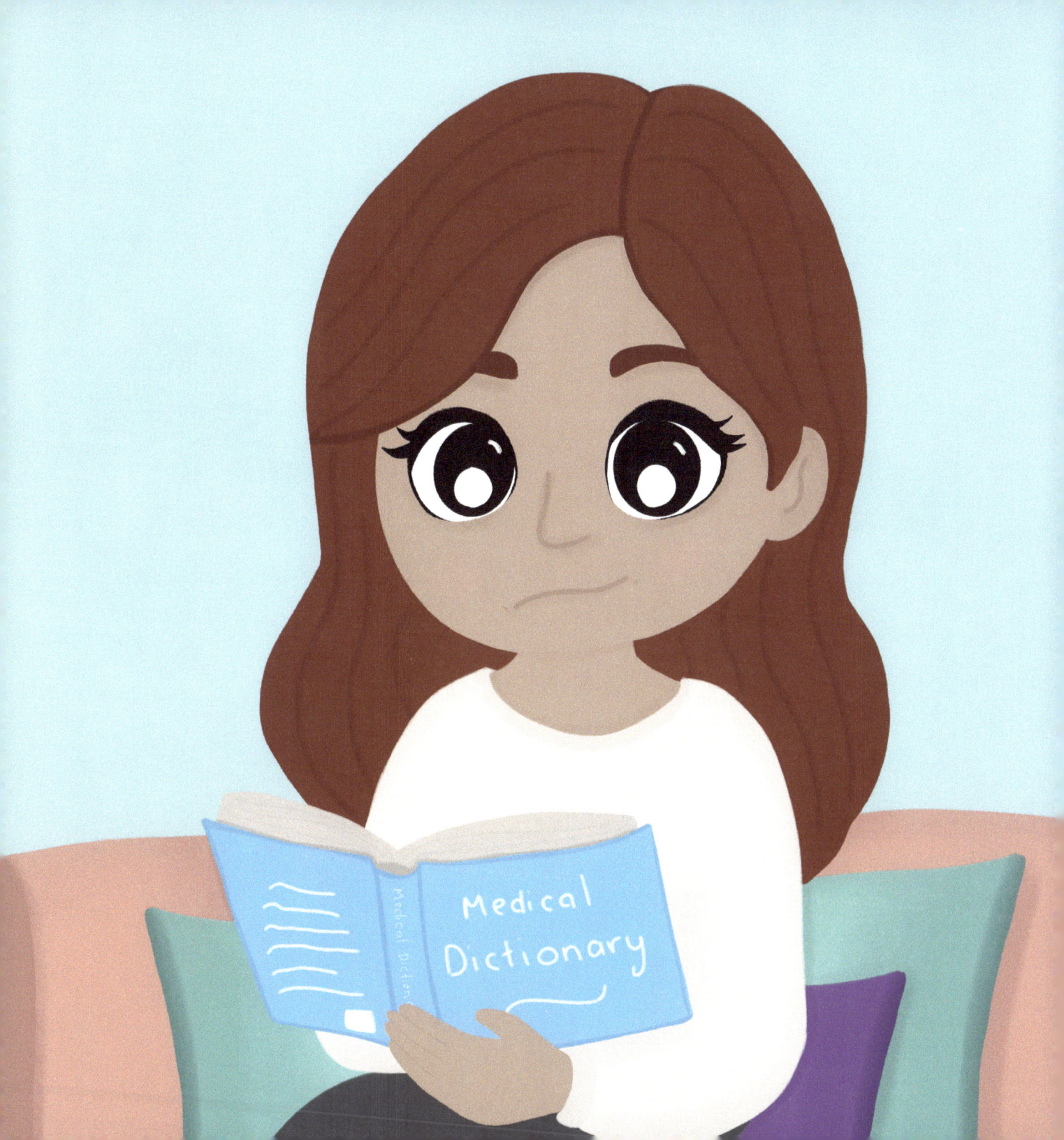

All the extra skills you've gained.
Though, you wish you never
had to.

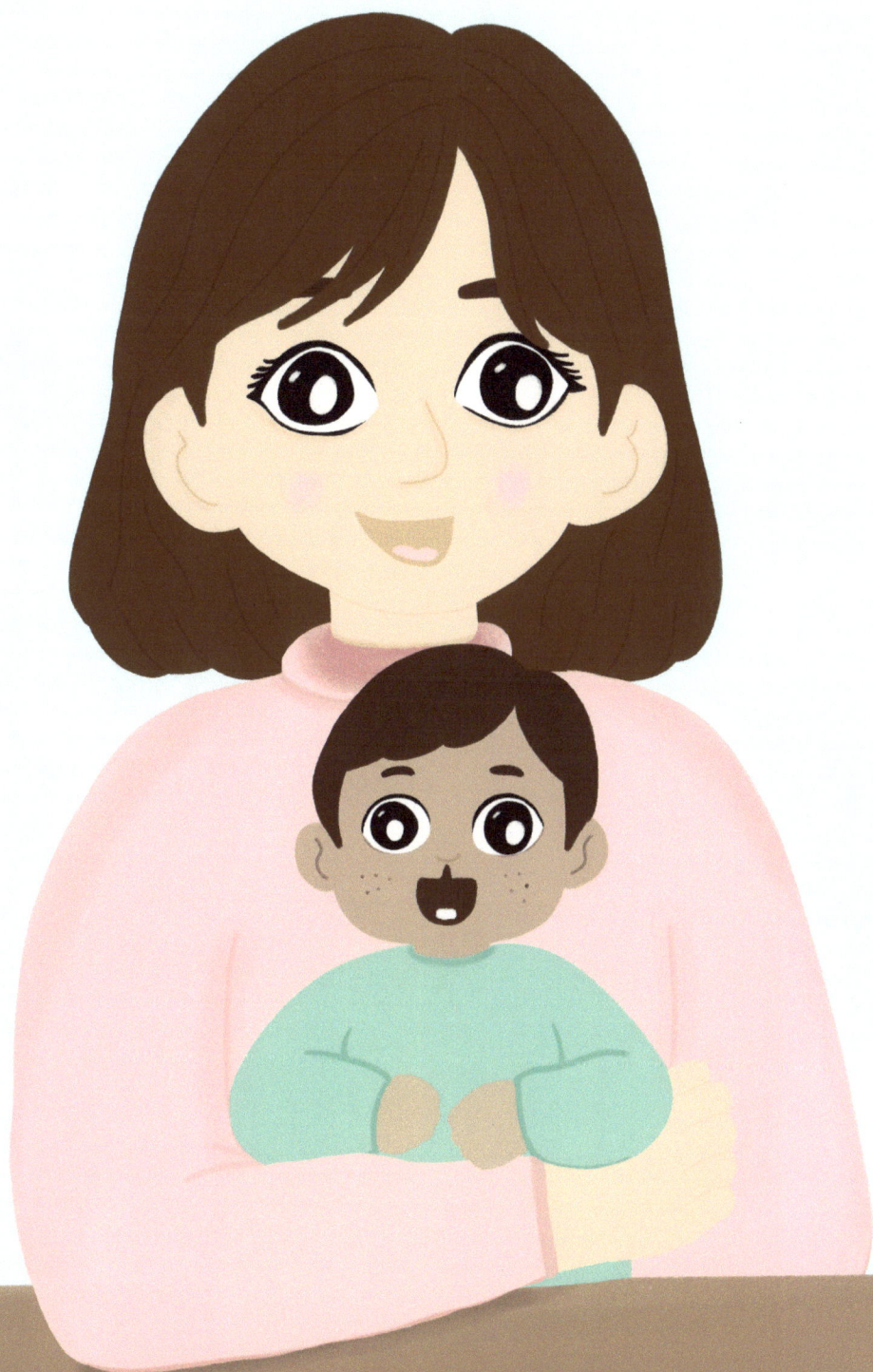

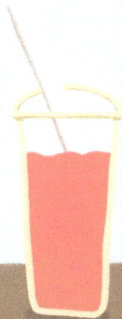

You're so brave,

Medical Mama.

Even when you don't feel it.

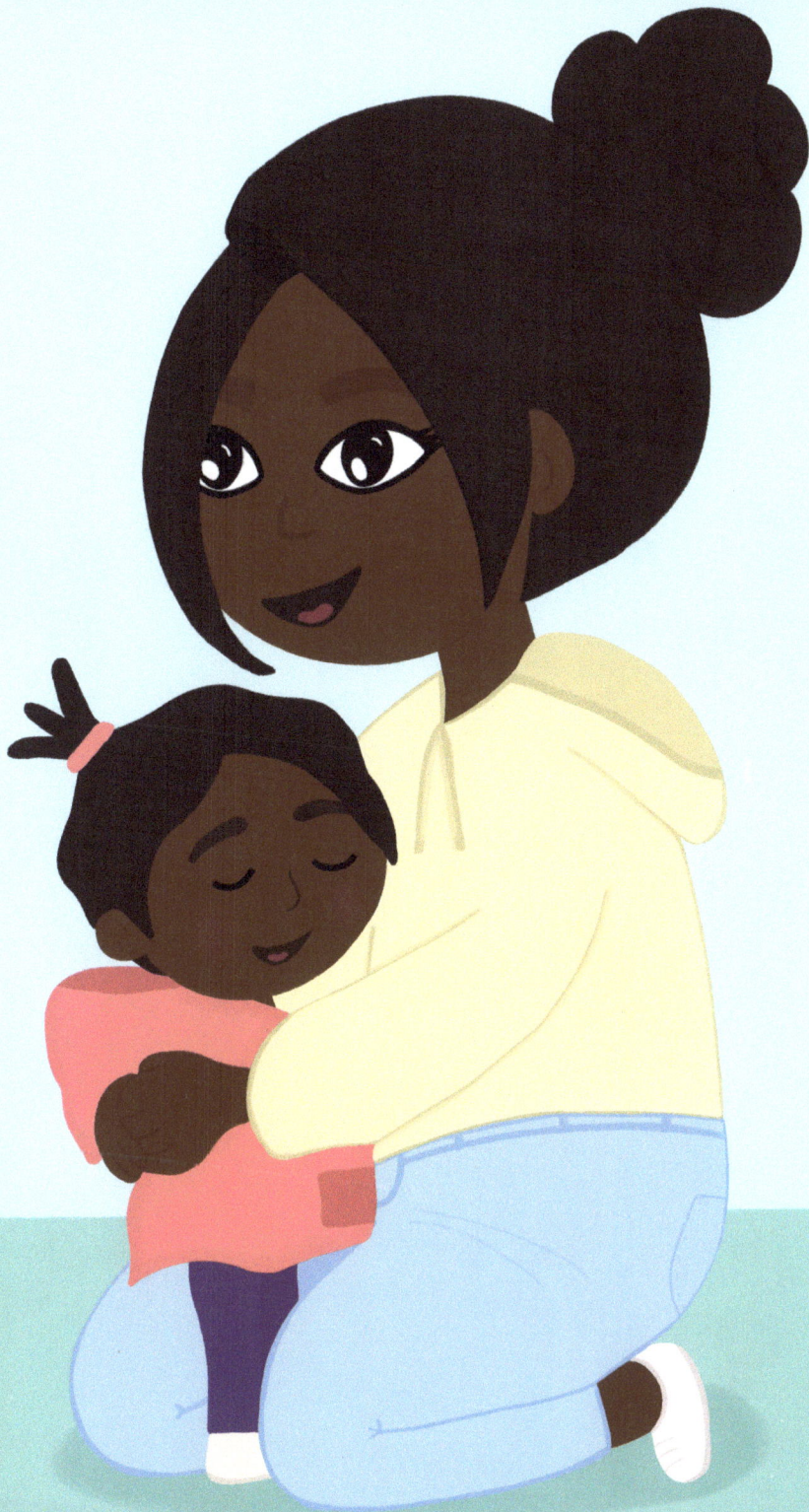

The heartbreak is real as you leave the hospital.
Your little one, still there, being cared for by others.

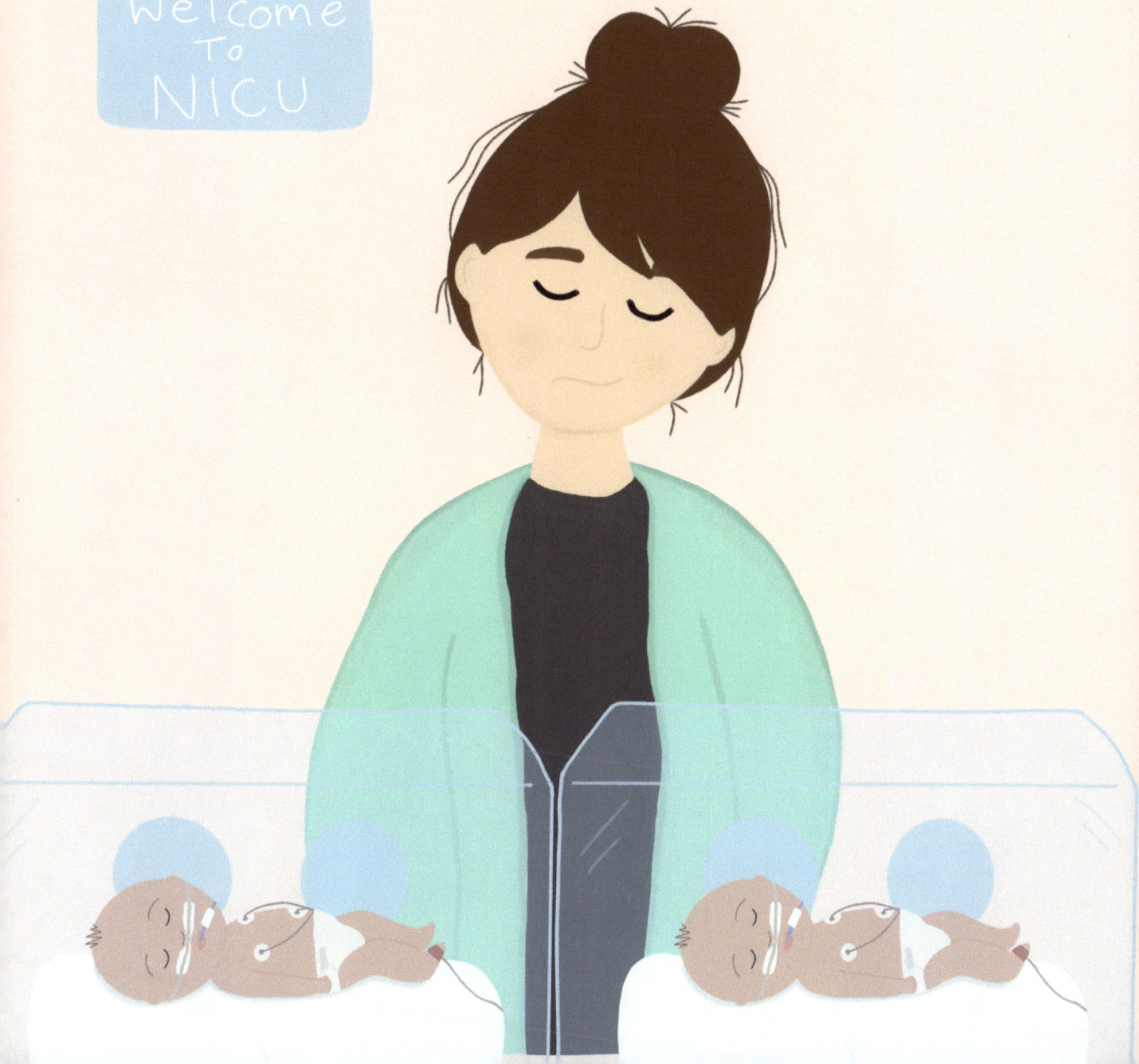

The surgeries are terrifying.
Nothing can quite prepare you.

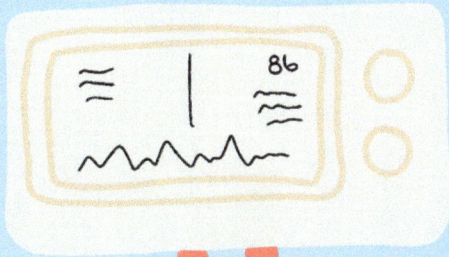

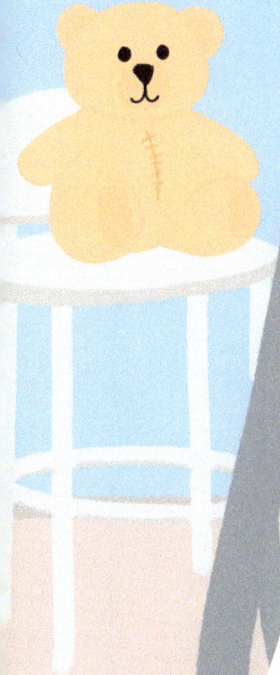

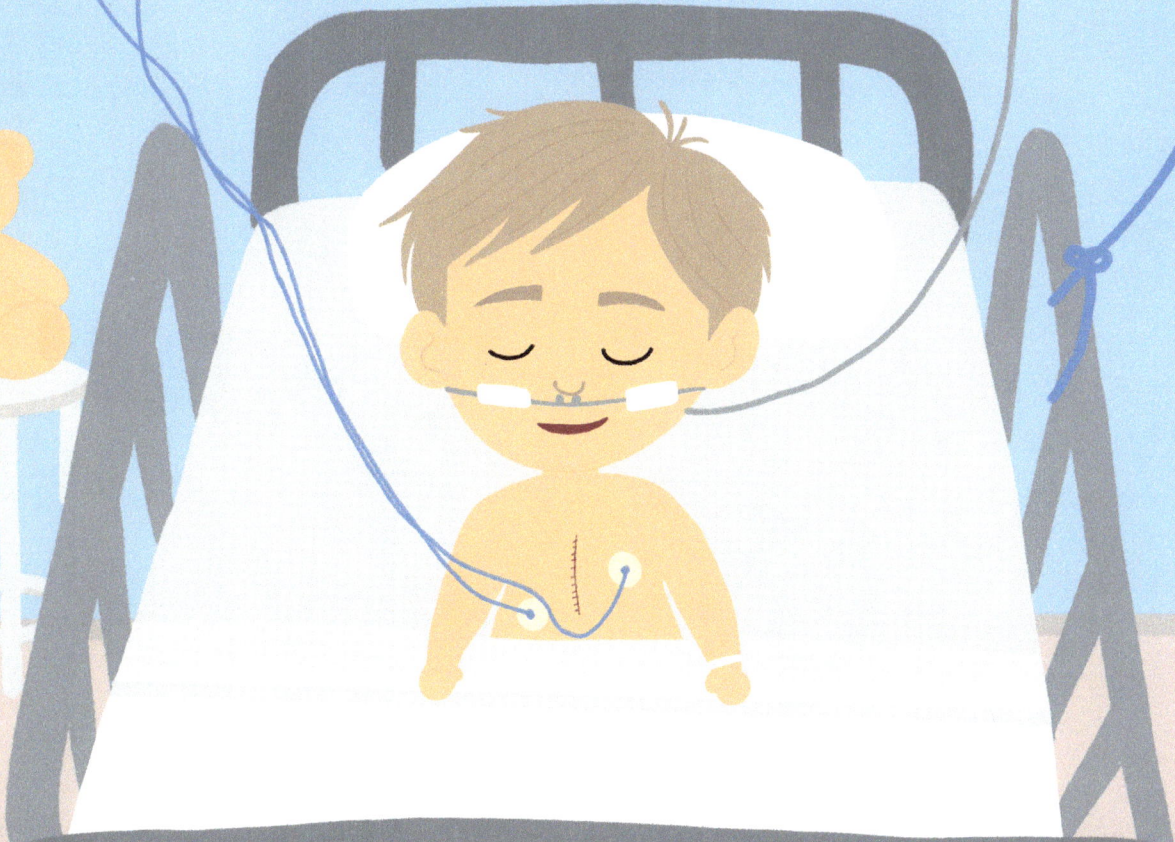

The exhaustion is draining.
Not even caffeine can fix it.

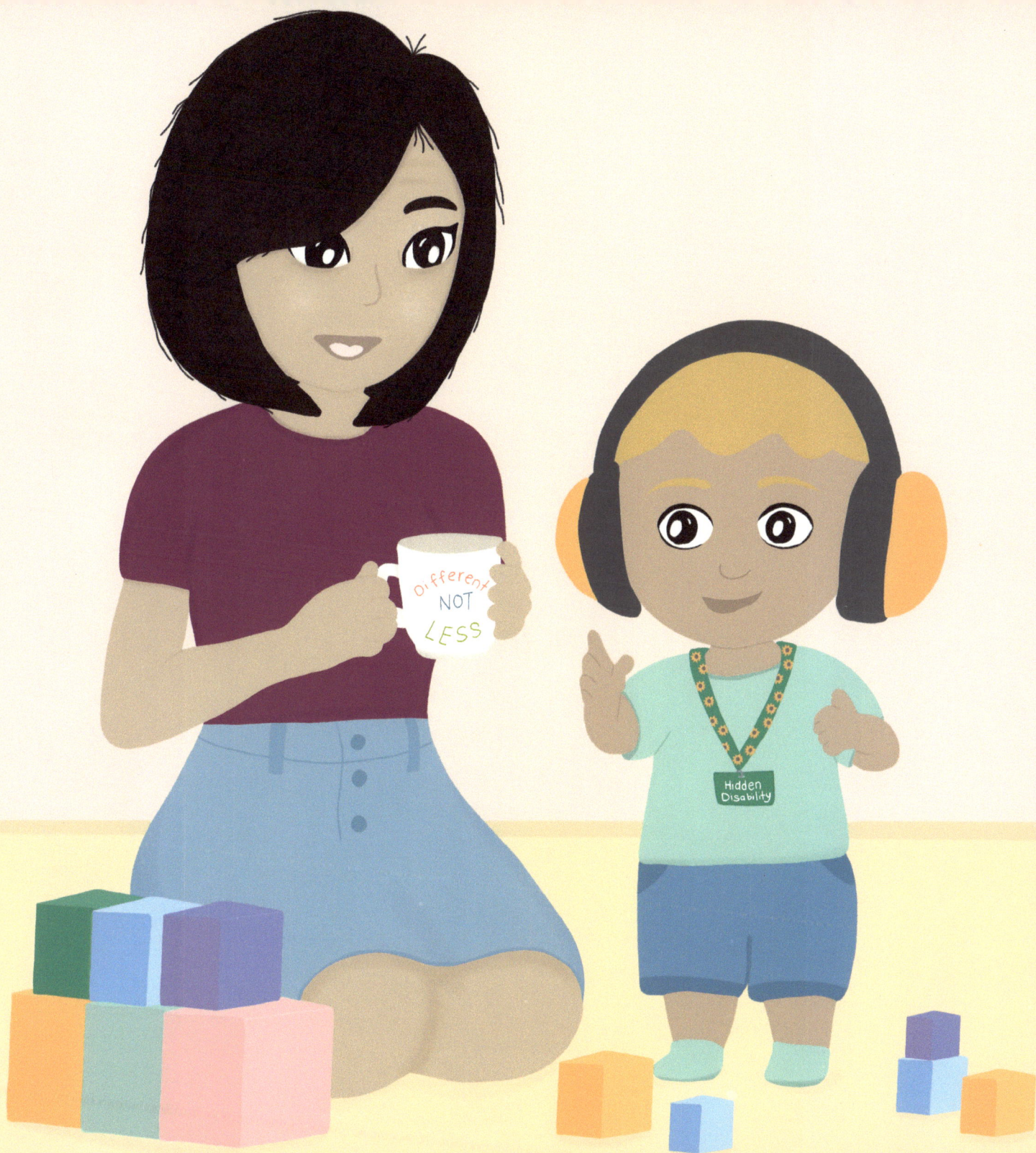

It's hard to see beyond the reality you're living now.

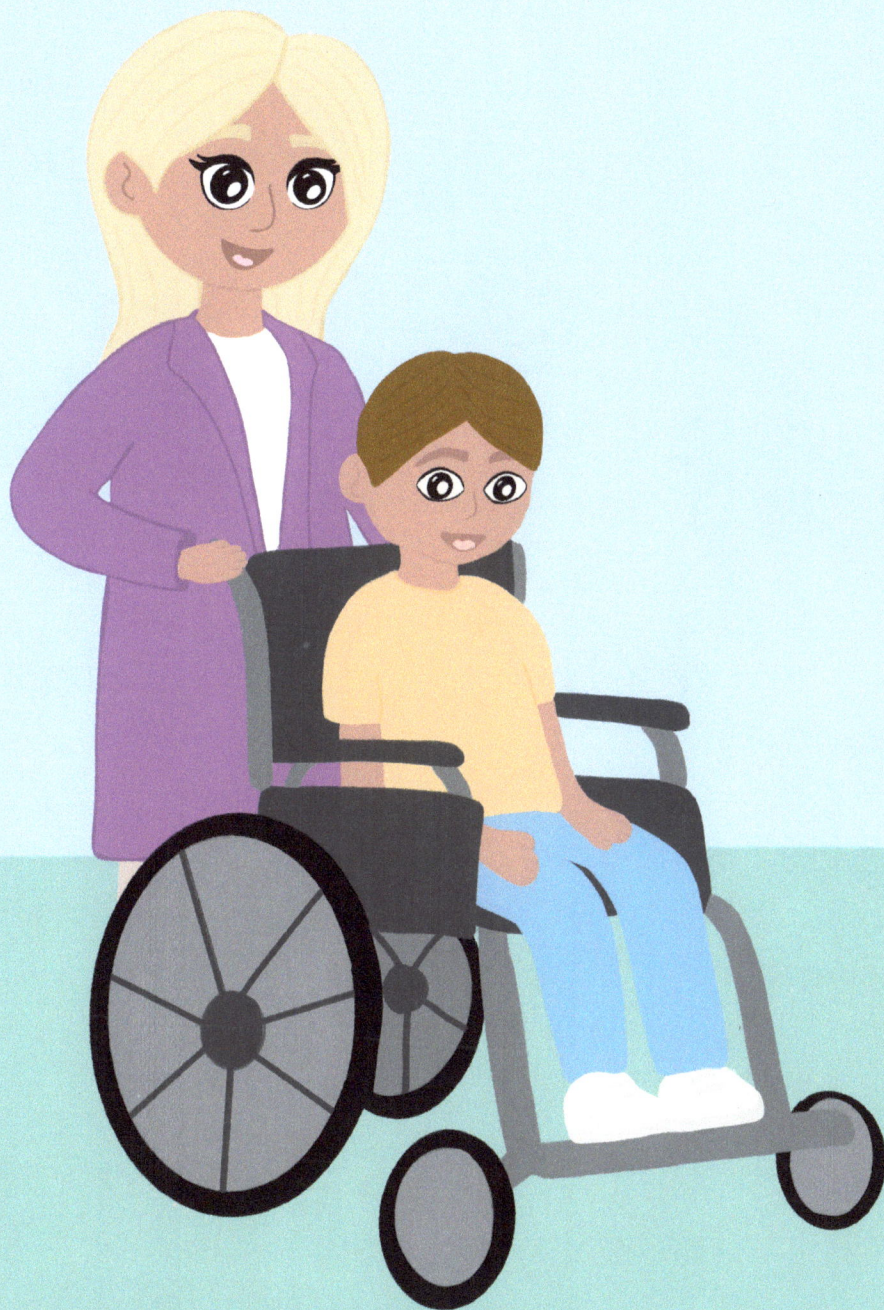

Hang in there,

Medical Mama.

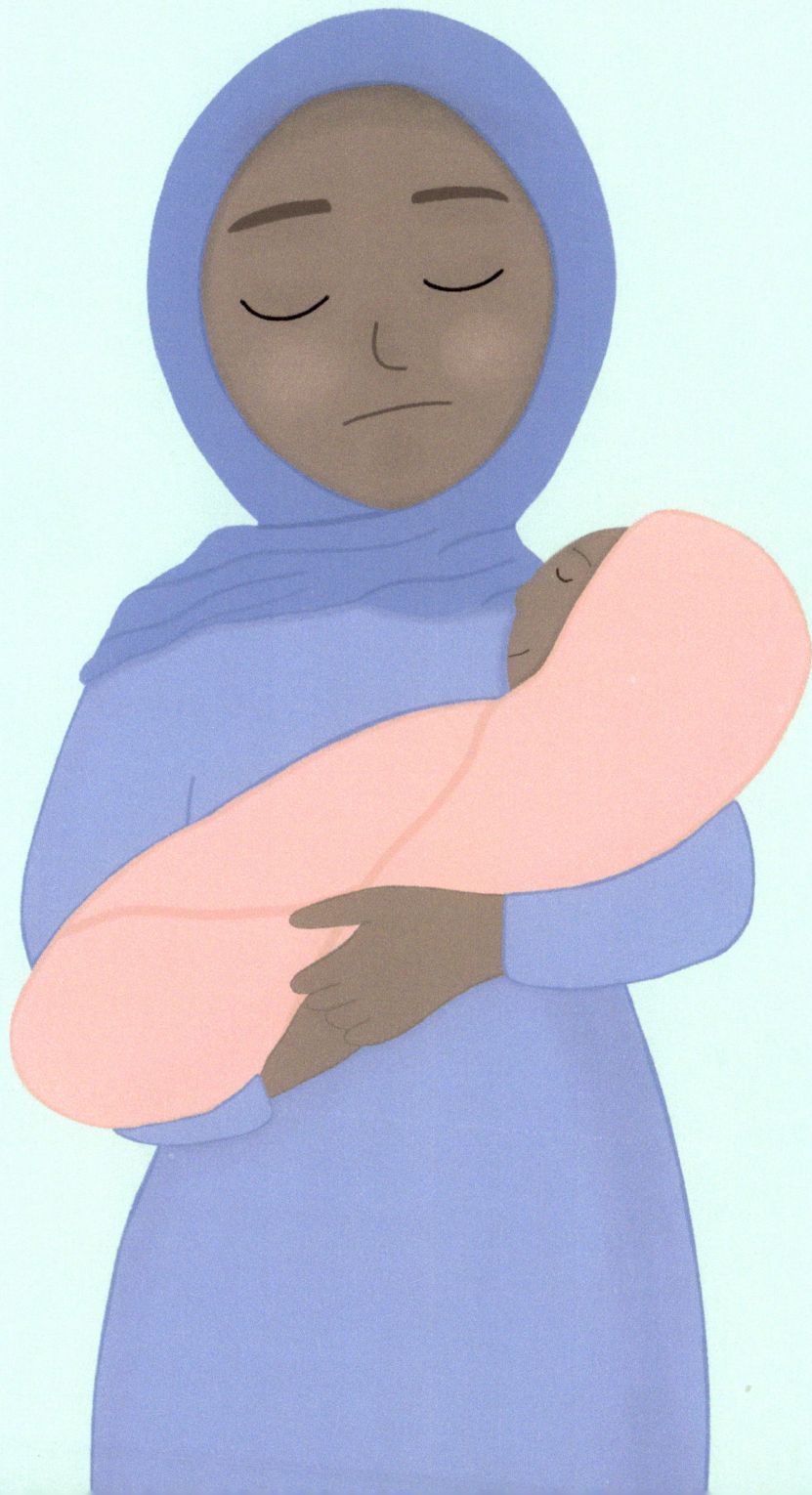

Because they are so worth it!

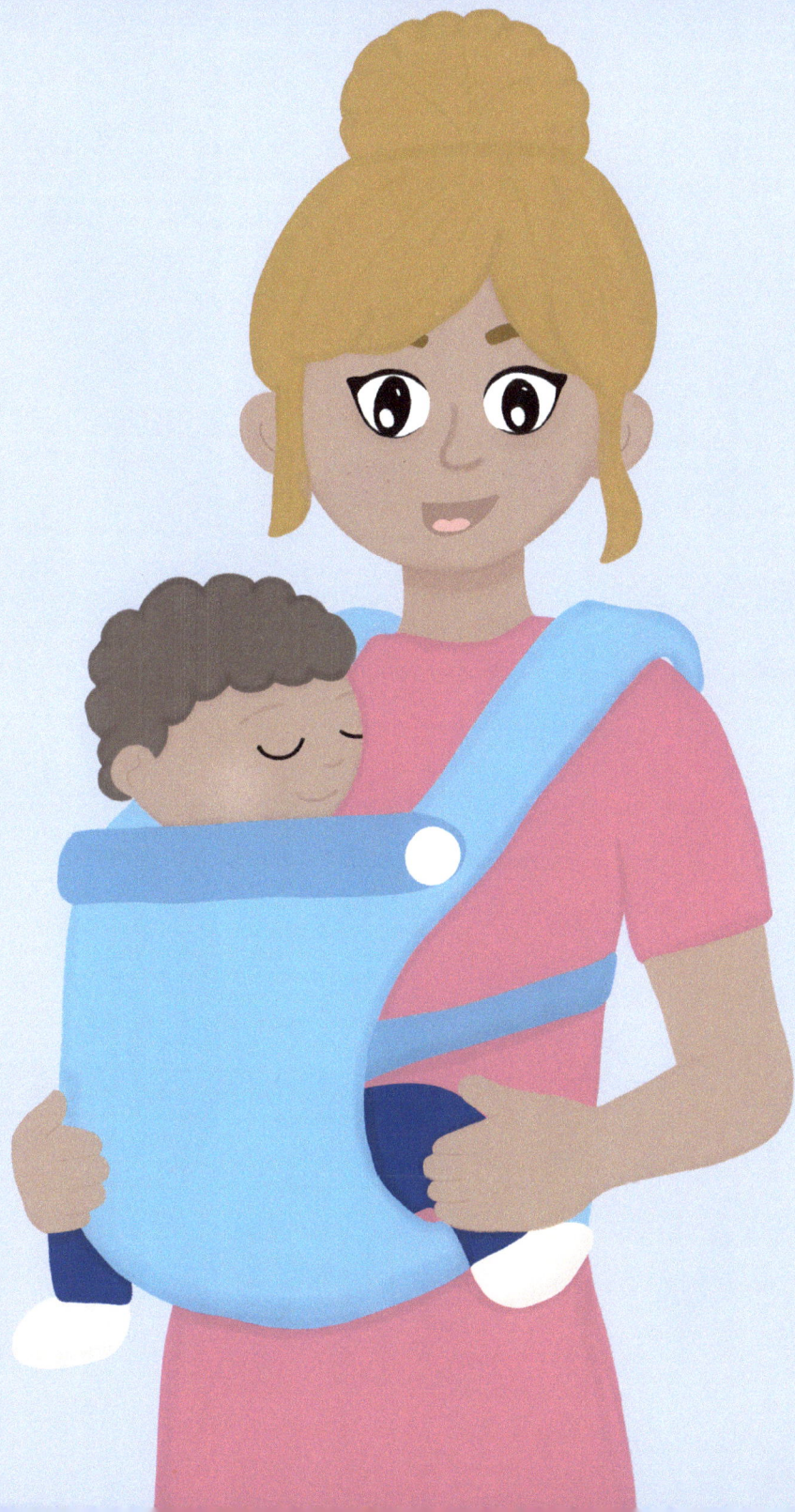

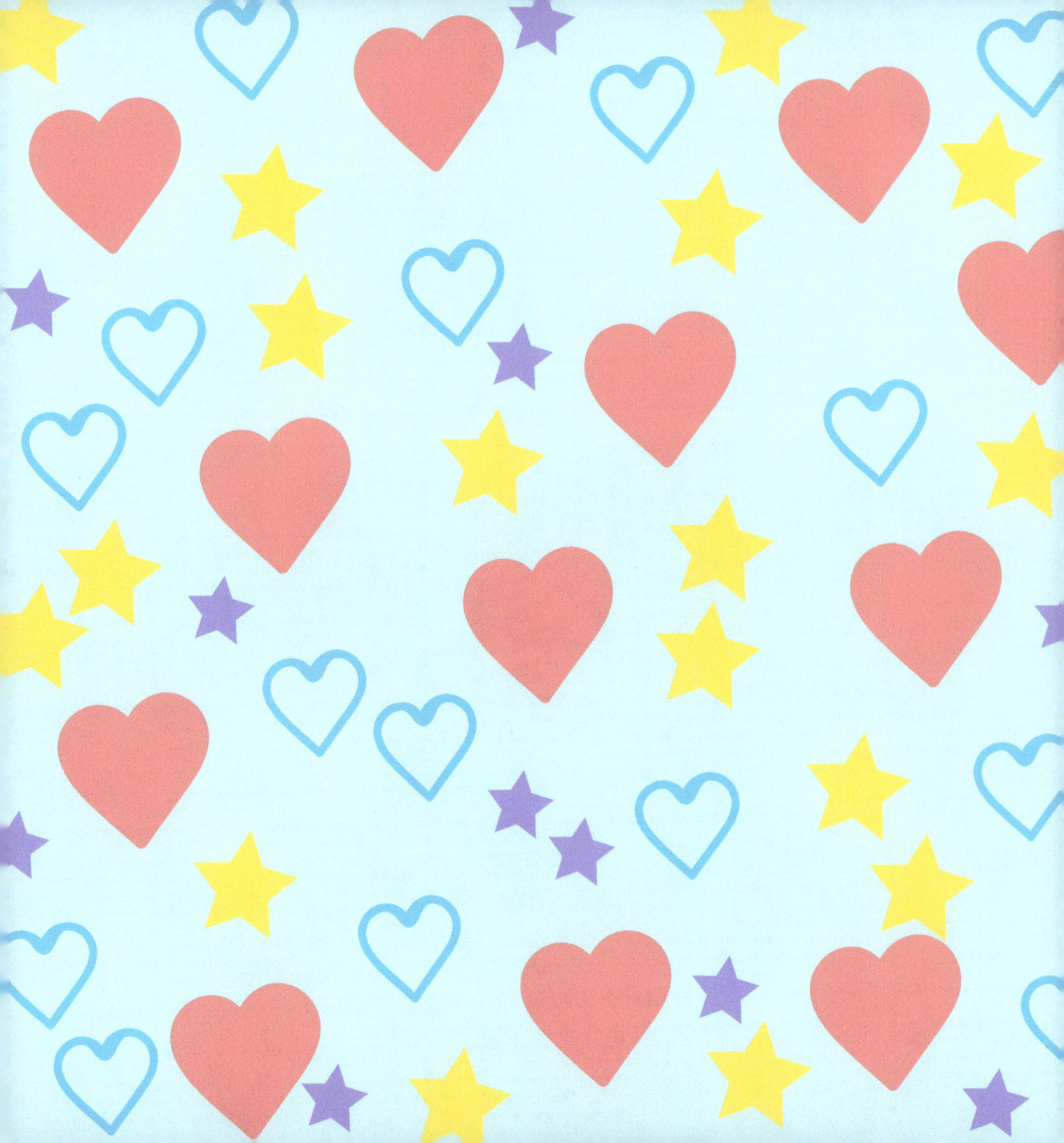

www.ingramcontent.com/pod-product-compliance
Lightning Source LLC
Chambersburg PA
CBHW041547260326
41914CB00016B/1571

9 781763 563445